Understanding

GN00360308

INDIGESTION
& ULCERS

Sigrid M. Burridge
& Dr Kenneth G. Wormsley

Published by Family Doctor Publications Limited
in association with the British Medical Association

IMPORTANT

This book is intended to supplement the advice given to you by your doctor. The authors and publisher have taken every care in its preparation. In particular, information about drugs and dosages has been thoroughly checked. However, before taking any medication you are strongly advised to read the product information sheet accompanying it. Your pharmacist will be able to help you with anything you do not understand.

© Family Doctor Publications 1993, 1995
Reprinted 1994
Second edition 1995

Medical Editor: Dr Tony Smith
Cover Artist: Colette Blanchard
Design: Create Publishing Services, Bath
Printing: Cambus Litho, Scotland, using acid-free paper

ISBN: 1 898205 02 7

Contents

CONTROL HEARTBURN LIKE NEVER BEFORE

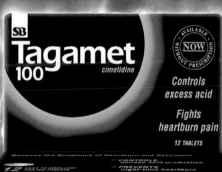

SB
Tagamet
100 *cimetidine*

• AVAILABLE • NOW • WITHOUT PRESCRIPTION •

Controls excess acid

Fights heartburn pain

12 TABLETS

Relieves the Symptoms of Heartburn and Dyspepsia

12 EASY TO SWALLOW COATED TABLETS
• CONTROLS excess acid production
• PREVENTS night-time heartburn

Tagamet 100
12 TABLETS
Controls excess acid - Fights heartburn pain

Now, thanks to the innovation of Tagamet 100 you can control heartburn like never before.

The conventional treatment of excess stomach acid – the cause of heartburn and indigestion – simply relies on its neutralisation. But Tagamet 100 works in a completely different way, by actually controlling excess acid production to keep it away for longer than an antacid.

It's not surprising that the breakthrough idea beh[...] Tagamet 100 led to the Nobel Prize for Medicine, gi[...] its dynamic new way of controlling heartburn.

Millions of sufferers have already felt the benefi[...] Tagamet 100's active ingredient and now you too can [...] the benefit by asking your pharmacist for Tagamet [...] which is now available without a prescription.

TAGAMET 100 ECLIPSES THE PAIN OF HEARTBUR[N]

ASK YOUR PHARMACIST

Contains cimetidine • Always read the label

Introduction

Indigestion (or dyspepsia) is a term used to describe complaints that seem to come from the part of the digestive tract connected with the eating and processing of food.

This book describes some of the most common causes of indigestion, as well as the tests that are required and the types of treatment that are available.

In addition, there are chapters about cancer of the stomach, inflammation of the stomach lining (gastritis), and non-ulcer dyspepsia, which is indigestion where no disease can be found after testing.

Patients with indigestion have upper abdominal discomfort or pain. There is often also a feeling of distension after food with an early feeling of being 'full up'. Other associated complaints include bloating, excess of wind with belching, regurgitation of food or gastric acid (the acid from the stomach), heartburn, lack of appetite, nausea and vomiting.

These complaints affect most people some of the time and many people much of the time. Indigestion affects patients repeatedly or continuously for weeks, months or even years. Often, these complaints are triggered by large meals or individual constituents of the food. However, the connection is

SYMPTOMS OF INDIGESTION

- Pain/discomfort in upper abdomen
- Heartburn
- Regurgitation of food or acid
- Bloating and excessive wind
- Rapid fullness after food & inability to eat a full meal
- Nausea/vomiting

not always easy to find because indigestion can occur during the night.

Most of us suffer from indigestion at some time and treat ourselves with medicines bought from the pharmacy. However, the indigestion is sufficiently bad to make one quarter of sufferers consult their general practitioner (GP). One of every hundred of the population visits the GP with food-related upper abdominal pain, and one in twenty of all GP consultations results from indigestion.

The manner in which these complaints occur can provide the doctor with a clue to an underlying disease. This is important, because the illness may require special treatment to produce a cure. In addition, if indigestion persists or recurs, or becomes progressively worse, or if treatment does not relieve symptoms, tests will be required. If it is possible to make a positive diagnosis from the test results, appropriate treatment becomes feasible, often with rapid relief of symptoms.

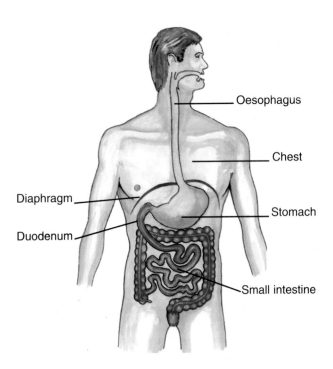

Oesophagus

Chest

Diaphragm

Stomach

Duodenum

Small intestine

The digestive tract.

Unfortunately, in more than half of all individuals with chronic indigestion, no cause for the indigestion is discovered. The complaints are then usually caused by disturbed function of the stomach or intestine. Negative tests for indigestion are very reassuring, because both the patient and the doctor know that no significant disease is present.

The illnesses that cause indigestion include oesophagitis (inflammation of the oesophagus, also called gullet or foodpipe); gastric ulcers (small wounds, often not bigger than half a little finger nail, in the

CAUSES OF INDIGESTION

- Oesophagitis
- Gastric ulcer
- Duodenal ulcer
- Cancer of the stomach
- Gastritis
- Non-ulcer dyspepsia

lining of the stomach); and duodenal ulcers (ulcers in the lining of the duodenum, which is the small intestine just beyond the outlet of the stomach).

Importance of lifestyle

Lifestyle plays an important part in the health and disease of the digestive system.

LIFESTYLE

The way in which we live (including our habits) has important effects on our health.

A number of abuses to which we subject ourselves and our digestive systems make it more likely that we will suffer from indigestion. If we can correct these self-inflicted injuries, we can often relieve the indigestion.

On the other hand, there are many causes of indigestion for which we are not responsible, so we must not make the problem worse by mistakenly feeling guilty about having brought it all on ourselves.

DIET

The main principle of healthy living is a balanced, all-round diet. Food should not contain too much fat, sugar or salt but should have sufficient roughage, vitamins and minerals. It is especially important to have an adequate intake of vitamin C, found in fresh fruit and green vegetables, and vitamin A (liver, dairy products and carrots) since normal amounts of these vitamins are necessary for defence against cancer.

Excessive food intake, or excessive consumption of individual dietary components, is undesirable. A large amount of food and drink during a meal encourages the regurgitation of food and gastric acid into the oesophagus, with damage to the lining of the oesophagus. Continued excessive food intake may result in superfluous body weight, which is not only a general health hazard but is also another of the causes of oesophagitis. An adequate intake of roughage in the form of whole-grain bread and fresh vegetables is desirable for the function of the bowels, but excessive consumption of roughage (in the form of added bran) may cause indigestion.

Food and drink should not be too hot, since excessively hot food may aggravate inflammation of the oesophagus or stomach.

FOOD INTOLERANCE

Some foodstuffs may directly injure the lining of the gut. For example, an excessive intake of salt may be a cause of gastric (stomach) ulcers. Similarly, eating a lot of pickles can cause inflammation of the lining of the oesophagus and the stomach.

Other foods injure the lining of the gut indirectly. For example, coffee, chocolate, peppermint, onions and fat cause indigestion by producing reflux of stomach contents into the oesophagus. Two thirds of the individuals who suffer from indigestion complain that their symptoms are made worse by drinking coffee. Interestingly, tea does not aggravate indigestion, so probably caffeine (which is present in both coffee and tea) is not the cause of the indigestion.

Allergic reactions

Allergic reactions to food occur in less than 1 per cent of adults and can also develop in children, especially those suffering from eczema

ALLERGIC REACTIONS TO FOOD

The human gut processes approximately 100 tons of food in a lifetime, but very few individuals develop food allergy. While the human gut is designed to defend the body against injury from bacteria, it usually avoids damaging reactions to food. Allergic reactions to food are rare.

and asthma. The foods that produce allergic reactions include nuts (especially peanuts), eggs, milk, fish, shell fish, soybeans and garlic. The allergic reactions can produce eczema or urticarial wheals (like nettle rash) in the skin, nasal congestion and asthmatic attacks with wheezing, as well as swollen and itching lips, or vomiting, cramps and diarrhoea. Sometimes the reaction is mild and insignificant but occasionally the affected individual may become very ill.

Some foods produce very well defined allergic reactions. For example, some children and adults react badly to wheat gluten, so that the intestine becomes inflamed and food cannot be digested properly. This condition is called coeliac disease, or sprue, and the allergy tends to be inherited. A quite different sort of indigestion is seen in some population groups who do not have the capacity to digest milk sugar (lactase deficiency). These patients develop discomfort, bloating, wind and sometimes diarrhoea if they drink a lot of milk. The condition is not a true allergy and has to be distinguished from the allergy to milk proteins from which babies occasionally suffer.

A few individuals react badly to food additives. It has been estimated that three people out of 10,000 do so in the UK. The proportion may be higher in children with eczema or asthma. Allergy-producing additives include tartrazine and synthetic colours, or preservatives (such as benzoates or sulphites).

However, in general, the concern about allergic reactions is greatly exaggerated, because food allergy is really quite rare.

FOODS THAT MAY PRODUCE ALLERGIC REACTIONS

- Nuts – especially peanuts
- Dairy products
- Fish – including shell fish
- Soybean products
- Garlic
- Cereals – especially wheat and rye
- Food additives

TESTING FOR FOOD ALLERGY

About one in four people believe that they react adversely to some foods. However, most of these reactions cannot be reproduced when the affected individuals are tested 'double-blind' – that is, when the food is disguised so that neither the patient nor the doctor knows what is being tested.

Food allergy test

When food intolerance is suspected, it is best to try the effect of an elimination (exclusion) diet followed by challenge with the food to be tested. This type of test involves eating a basic diet for two weeks and recording in a diary all the food eaten.

Food that is permitted includes fresh or frozen meat and poultry, white fish, fresh vegetables (e.g. lettuce, cabbage, sprouts and carrots), non-citrus fruits (e.g. apples, plums and peaches) and fruit juices (e.g. apple, pineapple and tomato) and rice and tapioca. Tinned or other processed foods should be avoided, since this type of food usually contains additives like colourings and preservatives.

Food items can then be reintroduced, one at a time every week or so, if there is no recurrence of any of the complaints. If symptoms do develop, the test should be repeated to exclude coincidence.

FOODS TO BE AVOIDED INITIALLY

- Tinned or processed meats (e.g. bacon, sausages & paté)
- Tinned or smoked fish & shellfish
- Potatoes, onions, cucumber & legumes (peas, beans & lentils)
- Citrus fruits, fruit juices & squashes
- Nuts
- Cereals (wheat, rye, oats & corn)
- Dairy products (milk, cream, butter, cheese & yoghurt)
- Eggs
- Coffee, tea & chocolate

DIET AND ULCERS

There has been a great deal of discussion about the role of diet in causing ulcers. It seems that there are factors in our diet which can cause ulcers and other factors which protect against ulcers. For example, too much salt may result in the development of gastric ulcers. Consumption of a lot of alcohol, coffee or cola drinks – especially when young – may increase the risk of duodenal ulcers, as does deficiency of fibre or protein in the diet.

SMOKING

Smoking aggravates heartburn, because it increases reflux of acid, a symptom of oesophagitis, from the stomach into the oesophagus. Smoking relaxes the muscles guarding the lower oesophagus and also slows the rate at which food is emptied from the oesophagus into the stomach.

In addition, smoking increases the likelihood of developing gastric or duodenal ulcers. The more cigarettes smoked, the greater the risk of ulcer disease. In addition, smoking delays the healing of ulcers and increases the risk of recurrence after healing. The risk of dying from an ulcer is six times greater in smokers than in non-smokers!

SMOKING AND ULCERS

- Smoking delays healing of ulcers
- The more cigarettes smoked, the longer ulcers take to heal
- Smoking interferes with ulcer-healing treatment
- Smoking increases the likelihood of ulcer relapse

INDIGESTION-PRODUCING DRUGS

A wide variety of drugs may directly damage the lining of the oesophagus. Injury usually begins within a few days of starting the drug treatment. Antibiotics are responsible for over half of the episodes of oesophagitis caused by drugs but iron pills, vitamin C, aspirin, drugs used for the treatment of arthritis and rheumatism and many others can also cause oesophageal inflammation.

DRUG-INDUCED OESOPHAGITIS

Oesophagitis caused by drugs can happen at any age. It is especially likely to occur if tablets or capsules are washed down with too little fluid or taken just before going to bed.

Patients with oesophagitis should always take tablets with food (unless instructed otherwise) or wash them down with at least a whole glass of water and then wait for at least 30 minutes before lying down. Patients suffering from oesophagitis should take any drugs needed for treatment in liquid or soluble form, if possible.

Drugs may also cause inflammation and ulcers of the lining of the stomach and duodenum. Even a single dose of aspirin can produce gastritis (inflammation of the stomach) and small gastric ulcers in all of us.

Other drugs used in the treatment of arthritis and rheumatism (or

DRUGS THAT MAY CAUSE OESOPHAGITIS

- Antibiotics
- Iron pills
- Vitamin C
- Aspirin
- Antirheumatic drugs

sometimes used inappropriately to relieve headache or menstrual pain) also produce ulcers. The amount of injury from aspirin and antirheumatic drugs is greatest during the first week of treatment and then tends to decrease.

Approximately 25% of all patients who attend arthritis clinics and continuously take large doses of aspirin or other antirheumatic drugs suffer from a gastric ulcer. However, the frequency of ulcers is less if the doses of these drugs are low. Aspirin and antirheumatic drugs should therefore be avoided if possible and other types of pain-killing drugs should be used to relieve pain.

If you require any further information on more appropriate drugs to take for pain relief, you should consult your GP or pharmacist. If anti-inflammatory drugs are required for the treatment of a rheumatic disorder, the dose should be the lowest that can control the complaints.

STRESS

The adverse effects of stress on the digestive system have been demonstrated in a number of excellent studies. Factors such as increased age, male gender and being unmarried increase the likelihood of stress and indigestion. The stress levels associated with personal problems are shown in the following table.

Evidence that stress may cause ulcers is shown by the fact that ulcers became a more serious problem during the heavy air raids of World War II. A more recent peacetime example of a stressful situation is provided by the frequent occurrence of ulcers among the immigrant 'guest' workers in central European countries.

Since too much stress has a serious effect on our health and well-being, as well as aggravating indigestion, it is important to seek expert advice. For example, if you have serious financial problems you should consult experts like a bank manager or a lawyer, or go to the Citizens' Advice Bureau. They can usually help to sort out financial affairs. If there are problems at work, a move to a different department or perhaps even a job elsewhere may help. Since some problems cannot be solved (for example bereavement, illness or even the behaviour of others), help yourself by worrying less. Start up a hobby that takes your mind off your problems; get a pet; and go out to make new friends.

It may even be that the indiges-

LIFE EVENTS AND STRESS

- **Highest stress factors**
  Death of spouse
  Death of close family
    member
  Divorce
  Marital separation
  Jail term
  Personal injury or illness
  Loss of job

- **High stress factors**
  Change in health of family
    member
  Fear of cancer
  Sex difficulties
  Business readjustment
  Financial difficulties

- **Moderate stress factors**
  Spouse begins or stops
    work
  Change in living conditions
  Son or daughter leaving
    home
  Trouble with in-laws
  Trouble with boss

tion itself is a stress. It is common to worry that one's illness is very serious. These fears may be exaggerated to such an extent that they become irrational and actually harmful. Seek advice from your doctor who will be able to arrange tests that reassure you.

KEY POINTS

Diet
✓ Balanced and not excessive

Smoking
✓ May aggravate all types of indigestion

Drug treatments
✓ Pain killers like aspirin and other antirheumatic drugs may cause indigestion

Stress
✓ Identify problem and seek help

Oesophagitis

The oesophagus is the tube leading from the mouth through the chest into the stomach. The wall of the oesophagus is made up of muscle that propels food into the stomach. Inside the muscle layer is a lining that becomes inflamed when it is injured by swallowed chemicals (like drugs prescribed for some other illness) or, more frequently, when stomach contents regurgitate into the oesophagus.

There are three main reasons for abnormally great amounts of stomach contents in the oesophagus. Firstly, there is an abnormal amount of reflux from the stomach because the muscles around the lower end of the oesophagus (called the 'lower oesophageal sphincter') relax too often. Normally, this muscle acts as a valve to prevent the contents of the stomach being regurgitated into the oesophagus. This muscle relaxes when a person

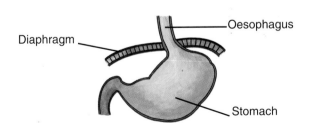

Diaphragm

Oesophagus

Stomach

Junction of normal oesophagus and stomach.

swallows but in patients with oesophagitis, the lower oesophageal sphincter relaxes for no obvious reason.

Alternatively, the lower oesophageal sphincter may be slack and incompetent because the muscle is infiltrated with fat in obese individuals, or because part of the stomach has slipped into the chest through the diaphragm (hiatal hernia).

When there is a hiatal hernia, the valve action at the lower end of the oesophagus cannot work properly. The inflammation, in turn, causes further weakening of the muscles surrounding the lower oesophagus, so that a vicious circle results.

A second reason for excessive reflux is because food stays in the stomach longer than normal. There is delay in the emptying of food from the stomach in approximately half of the patients with oesophagitis. Thirdly, the muscular wall of the oesophagus seems to function

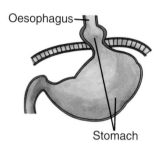

Hiatal hernia.

abnormally in many patients with oesophagitis. Normally, when there are regurgitated stomach contents in the oesophagus, the oesophageal muscle pushes these materials back into the stomach.

In patients with oesophagitis, this propulsion is defective, permitting prolonged contact between regurgitated gastric acid and the lining of the oesophagus. These muscle problems are aggravated when inflammation of the oesophagus becomes established.

GASTRO-OESOPHAGEAL REFLUX

Gastro-oesophageal reflux (regurgitation of stomach contents) causes oesophagitis when the amount refluxed is too great and the duration is too long. In other words, when acid and pepsin (a digestive ferment) produced by the stomach are in contact with the oesophageal lining for an excessively long period of time.

HOW COMMON IS OESOPHAGITIS?

At least twenty-five per cent of carefully studied patients with indigestion are found to suffer from oesophagitis. It has been estimated that about one in fourteen individuals suffer from daily heartburn. Nearly fifty per cent complain of at least one attack each month. Oesophagitis, which causes the heartburn, is therefore a common problem.

SYMPTOMS

The symptoms of oesophagitis do not correspond well with the degree of inflammation of the lining of the oesophagus. Thus, in at least fifty per cent of all patients who complain of oesophagitis, it is impossible to see inflammation during endoscopy (see page 15). Other types of test such as measurement of the amount of acidity in the lower oesophagus may be needed (see page 19).

These patients, without obvious oesophagitis, are said to suffer from gastro-oesophageal reflux disease. Apparently, the over-exposure to acid sensitizes the nerves of the oesophageal lining that feel pain, so that the feeling of discomfort precedes the visual and microscopic changes of inflammation. The alternative scenario is also true – some patients with very severe inflammation, and even ulceration, feel no discomfort at all. In other words, the symptoms of oesophagitis are very similar in most patients but the intensity of the complaint does not provide any guide to the amount of inflammation.

Regurgitation

Regurgitation of stomach contents, which fills the mouth with food or acid, may occur spontaneously or be brought on by stooping, straining or lying down. Regurgitated stomach contents may be present on the pillow in the morning.

Heartburn

As its name suggests, heartburn is the name given to a burning sensation or discomfort behind the breastbone and in the upper abdomen under the ribs. Heartburn (also called pyrosis) is a symptom that affects approximately two-thirds of patients with oesophagitis. The discomfort varies in severity and duration and is often made worse by lying down, stooping, on exertion after meals and by factors that increase pressure in the abdomen, such as pregnancy. Heartburn is also

FACTORS THAT INCREASE HEARTBURN

- Lying down
- Stooping
- Exertion after meals
- Repeated vomiting
- Aerophagy
- Increased pressure in abdomen (e.g. pregnancy)
- Hot food and drink
- Components of diet

caused, or aggravated, by repeated vomiting and by aerophagy (a bad habit that involves swallowing air and belching).

Heartburn may also be directly aggravated by meals, especially by food or drink at too high a temperature; by eating food, like muesli, which can 'scratch' the lining of the inflamed oesophagus; by citrus fruits such as oranges, lemons and grapefruit; by acidic substances like vinegar; by spicy foods such as chillies and curries; or by drinking alcoholic beverages. Alternatively, heartburn is made worse by foods that promote reflux from the stomach. These include foods containing large amounts of fat (such as pies, pizzas, pastries and some breakfast cereals); chocolate; peppermint (which is surprising, since so many indigestion remedies include peppermint); and onions (which contain chemicals that cause reflux). In addition, coffee but not tea promotes reflux, as does smoking.

Pain

Continuous or spasmodic pain in the upper abdomen, in the middle just below the ribs, or behind the breastbone, is suffered by about one-third of patients with oesophagitis. The pain may be caused or made worse by swallowing and is usually the result of spasm of the oesophageal muscles.

Less frequently, oesophageal pain is caused by the development of an ulcer or ulcers, similar to the ulcers of the stomach and duodenum and also caused by regurgitation of gastric acid.

Difficulty in swallowing

Patients suffering from severe reflux may have problems with swallowing foodstuffs. This complaint is also called 'dysphagia'; it is a serious symptom that always requires a visit to the doctor. At first, difficulty may be experienced with solids only, but later also with liquids. The food fails to pass into the stomach normally, producing a distressing sensation of sticking on the way down behind the breastbone. Some patients with swallowing difficulties may have a normal sized oesophagus but mostly the oesophagus is narrowed by scarring from inflammation or a healed ulcer.

FOODS THAT AGGRAVATE HEARTBURN

- Coarse foods
- Citrus fruits
- Acidic substances
- Spicy foods
- Alcoholic beverages
- Foods rich in fat
- Chocolate
- Peppermint
- Onions
- Coffee

SYMPTOMS OF REFLUX FROM THE STOMACH

- Regurgitation
- Heartburn
- Pain
- Difficulty in swallowing
- Bleeding
- Wheezing, etc.
- Sore throat, hoarseness, etc.

Bleeding

As a result of severe inflammation, the lining of the oesophagus may be very susceptible to injury from poorly chewed food. Consequently, bleeding may occur and is usually not noticed unless there is quite a lot, when the blood may be vomited. Sometimes the bleeding is slight but persistent. In this case the patient may not notice that anything is wrong until he or she develops symptoms of anaemia.

Throat and chest complaints

Many patients with oesophagitis wake at night coughing, choking and spluttering, having inhaled some stomach contents into the lungs. This night-time wheezing is often accompanied by early morning hoarseness and a feeling of a lump in the throat. Heartburn and other symptoms usually associated with oesophagitis may be minimal or absent. Some patients can develop more serious problems. For example, a sore throat in the morning may become chronic and be associated with chronic laryngitis and hoarseness. A few individuals even develop erosions of the back molar teeth. More importantly, some patients with reflux troubles can develop 'gastric asthma', with asthmatic attacks occurring at night, at times of the year when allergic asthma (related to the amount of pollen in the air) does not occur. There is also an increased likelihood of bronchitis. Patients with gastric asthma may benefit greatly from anti-reflux treatment even when reflux is not an obvious problem.

TESTS AND INVESTIGATIONS

Endoscopy

Endoscopy is a procedure in which a flexible tube, about the thickness of a little finger, is passed into the oesophagus and stomach and through the stomach into the duodenum. The tube is made up of fibre glass bundles which transmit a strong light from a light source outside the body to the end of the tube inside the gut. By means of a lens system, the inside of the gut can be studied and the view is made even better because the end of the endoscope can be bent in all directions by the doctor who is carrying out the test, using a very ingenious system of levers.

The procedure involves fasting from midnight, because there is no point in having an endoscopy if the stomach is full of food. On arrival in the endoscopy unit, the patient is usually interviewed by a nurse, who notes details about the individual and his or her past and present illnesses on a form. The doctor later records the endoscopic findings on the same form. The procedure is explained in detail to the patient who is then asked to sign a form consenting to the endoscopy,

INVESTIGATIONS

One or several tests may be required if a patient suffers from indigestion. The tests are needed to confirm the doctor's diagnosis, to establish the likely course of an illness, or to guide the treatment of the patient. The most important test for studying any part of the gut, but especially the upper part, is endoscopy. Endoscopy has replaced barium X-rays as the investigation that is likely to provide the most information.

because such consent is necessary for all procedures carried out in hospital. The patient then takes off outer clothing, puts on a hospital gown, takes out any dentures and

lies on a bed or stretcher that can be wheeled into the endoscopy suite. There, a doctor (usually assisted by a couple of nurses) will again describe what is going to happen during the endoscopy and will answer the patient's questions. The patient is then given an injection of a sedative, to make him or her drowsy and relieve any worries. If the patient wants to drive or go straight back to work, or if he or she has previously undergone an endoscopy, they can do without the injection and instead receive a local anaesthetic spray to the back of the throat. After this type of spray, it is best not to eat or drink for four hours since food may go down the 'wrong way'.

When the patient is drowsy, the doctor will insert a gag to prevent the patient biting the endoscope. The endoscope is then passed into the oesophagus, over the back of the tongue. There may be transient discomfort, with a feeling that one wants to be sick, but that feeling usually passes off quickly, especially if the patient remembers to pant, or breathe rapidly. Once the endoscope is in the oesophagus, it can be quickly pushed on into the stomach under direct vision. Any disease of the oesophagus can be recorded. In the stomach, the doctor may have to empty out gastric juice and bile, which can be done by using a suction channel in the endoscope. The endoscope also has a system for flushing water across the lenses in the tip of the instrument, to wash away any bile or mucus. Once in the stomach, the doctor will find the pylorus, which is the exit from the stomach into the duodenum. The duodenum is then entered and inspected. In the duodenum, the doctor will look especially for an ulcer, which is usually found within an inch or so of the pylorus. If the duodenal lining is normal, the endoscope is withdrawn into the stomach and the whole of the stomach is examined for inflammation, ulcers or cancer. Since the tip of the endoscope is so flexible that it can be bent back on itself, even the upper parts of the stomach can be seen.

In addition to obtaining a good look at the stomach, it is possible to pass a very small forceps down a channel in the endoscope. The forceps can be used to obtain specimens of the lining of the gut for later examination under a microscope if, for example, cancer is suspected. Other specimens can be used for culturing bacteria. The procedure by which such tiny specimens are obtained is called 'biopsy' and is usually quite painless. Any bleeding which occurs is usually slight and not much more than from a small cut on a finger.

After examining the stomach, the endoscope is withdrawn into the oesophagus, which can again be studied. The endoscope is then withdrawn from the mouth. After the endoscopy, the patient can sleep for a little while until the effect of the sedative wears off. He or she then receives a cup of tea and a biscuit (to make up for missing breakfast), is given the result of the test, and is collected by a relative or friend. It is recommended that patients do not drive a car, or handle machinery, and do not make any major decisions until the day after the endoscopy in case the sedative has impaired concentration.

The whole procedure, which is called oesophago-gastro-duodenoscopy (or 'gastroscopy' for short), takes ten to fifteen minutes when used for making a diagnosis. The patient is not usually unconscious and, indeed, sometimes actually follows the whole procedure through a viewing attachment on the endoscope or on a television screen since the endoscope can be linked to a video system. A visual and written record of the procedure and findings is filed in the patient's case notes.

Most patients have no trouble with endoscopy and because of the sedative many cannot even remember having the test done. Some may experience a sore throat. A few patients have trouble with swallowing the tube because the back of the throat is too sensitive. The endoscopy has then to be carried out under general anaesthetic, but this is necessary in only about one or two patients in a hundred.

Apart from a transient sore throat, complications are very uncommon. For example, patients occasionally bleed after a biopsy or, very rarely, the endoscope may perforate the gut – especially if there is obstructive disease of the oesophagus.

Endoscopy for oesophageal disease

Patients with upper abdominal pain or discomfort, or with heartburn or regurgitation, may be suffering from oesophagitis. If the complaints persist despite appropriate treatment for two to four weeks, or recur rapidly after treatment, the patient should be sent for endoscopic examination. The examination is usually arranged by the GP who sends the patient either directly for endoscopy (if there is a local 'open-access' endoscopy unit) or to the gastroenterologist (specialist in gut diseases) who will arrange the examination in his or her unit.

If the investigation shows inflammation or ulceration of the lower oesophagus, the diagnosis has been established. However, the doctor carrying out the endoscopy always goes on to examine the rest of the upper gut because, for example, the patient may also be suffering from an ulcer. Thus, it has been shown

ENDOSCOPY

Without doubt endoscopy is the most valuable tool for investigating indigestion since a diagnosis of 'disease' or 'no disease' can be made rapidly and accurately in most

that between one third and a half of patients with duodenal ulcer also suffer from oesophagitis.

About 50 per cent of the patients with heartburn or regurgitation have an endoscopically normal oesophagus. The doctor may then biopsy the lining of the oesophagus, because even normal looking oesophageal lining may show evidence of inflammation under a microscope. Alternatively, the doctor may arrange for a 24-hour measurement of the acidity in the oesophagus.

The other complaint that always requires endoscopy, usually as soon as the symptom is noticed, is dysphagia (when an individual feels that food sticks on the way down behind the breastbone). In a patient with this complaint, endoscopy often shows narrowing of the oesophagus and it may be impossible to push the endoscope through into the stomach. The doctor then always takes some biopsies for microscopic examination. If the biopsy tissue shows scarring and inflammation, the doctor subsequently stretches the narrowed oesophagus so that the passage becomes wider. On the other hand, if the patient is not suffering from oesophagitis but from cancer of the oesophagus (which usually shows itself with dysphagia) the biopsy will show the cancerous tissue and the patient will require surgery or radiotherapy.

Barium meal X-ray

When endoscopic examination is not quickly available, patients with indigestion with features suggestive of oesophageal disease are often sent for a barium meal X-ray. The examination is simple. A fasting individual drinks some barium suspension, which tastes chalky. As the patient swallows, the passage of the barium meal is followed from the mouth down the oesophagus and into the stomach. An ordinary barium meal is not very useful for confirming the diagnosis of oesophagitis. On the other hand, the narrowing that is causing swallowing difficulties is usually well shown, as is the length of the oesophagus that is narrowed. If narrowing is found by barium meal X-ray, an urgent endoscopy and biopsy must be carried out to obtain tissue for microscopic examination.

The doctor usually examines the patient not only in the upright position, but also when the barium is in the stomach. The patient lies down and the doctor may then press on the stomach to see whether there is a hiatal hernia (that is, whether part of the stomach slides up into the chest).

Measuring acidity in the oesophagus

To measure reflux of stomach contents, a small tube is inserted into the oesophagus. The tube has a special tip that can measure changes in the acidity of the contents (called 'pH-metry'). The tube is passed through the patient's nose into the oesophagus where it remains for 24 hours. The acidity measurements are automatically recorded on a small portable recorder the size of a 'Walkman'. A 'normal' person has occasional reflux of small amounts of acid stomach contents into the oesophagus, especially after a large meal and on exercise. This acid reflux is usually of short duration and does not cause any trouble. In patients with heartburn, the amount and duration of the acid reflux is abnormally great.

Measuring the rate of passage through the oesophagus and stomach

It is easy for the doctor to measure the rate at which food passes through the oesophagus and out of the stomach. The patient is asked to eat some food (such as scrambled eggs) injected with a very small amount of harmless radioactive material. The progress of the food is monitored as it passes through the oesophagus and the stomach. The investigation can confirm the slowing of the passage of food through the oesophagus and, indeed, food may actually stick and not move at all in some patients whose oesophageal muscle function is abnormal or has been severely damaged by reflux.

Using a similar technique, it is easy to measure the rate at which food and fluids leave the stomach. In about half of the patients with oesophagitis, stomach emptying is slowed (making food and acid available for regurgitation into the oesophagus for longer periods than normal).

TREATMENT

Change in lifestyle

It is necessary for patients with oesophagitis to change their lifestyle for the condition to improve. Meals should be small rather than large and, if necessary, more frequent to avoid overloading the stomach. It is also necessary to avoid very hot food or drink. The diet should be changed, so as to avoid the food items (see page 14) that aggravate heartburn. Evening meals should be eaten early, so that the stomach is empty at bedtime. At least four hours should be allowed after meals, and two hours after the last drink before lying down or going to bed.

TREATMENT OF OESOPHAGITIS

The treatment of patients with oesophagitis is designed to overcome the faults that cause oesophageal inflammation. Treatment decreases the regurgitation of acid from the stomach into the oesophagus and increases the clearance of regurgitated stomach contents from the oesophagus. Stomach emptying is also increased. In other words, it is necessary to improve the way that the muscles of the oesophagus and stomach function. It is also essential to decrease the amount of acid that the stomach produces. These aims are achieved by changing the lifestyle of the patient with oesophagitis and by using drugs.

Whenever possible, patients with oesophagitis should avoid wearing belts (braces are preferable), tight girdles and suspender belts. Stooping and heavy lifting are best avoided, especially after meals. Patients should attempt to lose weight if they are too fat. No tablets or capsules for any treatment should be taken within one hour of lying down. At night, it is often helpful to raise the head of the bed by about

COMBATING OESOPHAGITIS

- Eat small meals
- Avoid very hot food and drinks
- Avoid foods that aggravate heartburn
- Go to bed with an empty, dry stomach
- Avoid lying down immediately after meals; use a reclining chair instead
- Do not wear belts, girdles or suspender belts, if possible
- Avoid stooping and heavy lifting, especially after meals
- Lose weight, if too heavy
- Stop smoking
- Do not take any tablets or capsules less than one hour before lying down

20 cm (8 – 9 inches) or to use a firm wedge of similar height to raise the chest and head. This will help to drain the oesophagus and lessen the amount of reflux from stomach to oesophagus that occurs in patients with oesophagitis who are lying down. The bed can be raised on wooden blocks or bricks. Increasing the number of pillows does not usually help because the patient may slide off them during sleep. Smoking should be cut down or, better still, stopped altogether.

Treatment to improve muscle function

Patients with severe and persistent symptoms may derive additional benefit from 'prokinetic' drugs – drugs that improve the function of muscles. These drugs act to increase the strength of the lower oesophageal sphincter (which reduces reflux from the stomach). They also stimulate the muscles of the oesophagus to propel food down the oesophagus and also to increase the rate at which regurgitated stomach contents are expelled from the oesophagus. Prokinetic drugs also improve the function of the stomach so that food and acid are emptied more rapidly from the stomach into the small intestine. Prokinetic drugs include metoclopramide (*Maxolon*), domperidone (*Motilium*) and, most recently, cisapride (*Prepulsid* or *Alimix*). Treatment may have to continue for a few weeks or many months.

Treatment to reduce the amount of gastric acid

Two types of drugs are used to decrease the amount of gastric acid that is available for regurgitating from the stomach into the oesophagus. Antacids neutralize the acid that has already been secreted by the stomach. Alternatively, it is possible to use drugs that prevent the secretion of acid by the stomach lining.

Antacids

Antacids are usually the first line of treatment, as mild symptoms are often rapidly relieved by these preparations. These drugs work by neutralizing the acid produced by the stomach and are therefore taken as often as required. Most doctors prefer the type called raft antacids (such as *Gastrocote*, *Gaviscon* and *Topal*) which also contain material that makes the antacid float to the surface of the stomach contents. When the patient lies down or stoops the antacid 'raft' enters the oesophagus first and acts as a kind of ball valve.

Antacids by themselves do not control the symptoms of more severe oesophagitis, in part perhaps because antacid preparations cannot be swallowed during sleep, when much reflux occurs. In this type of situation, it becomes necessary to use more powerful drugs that inhibit the production of acidic gastric juice.

H_2-receptor antagonists

The H_2-receptor antagonists (see page 47) (cimetidine, ranitidine, nizatidine and famotidine) are drugs that have been used to treat oesophagitis for as long as 15 years.

These drugs are usually taken two to four times a day, an hour after meals, and the last dose at least two hours before going to bed. The drug is best taken in soluble or dispersible form, since tablets tend to stick for some time in the oesophagus of patients with oesophagitis. After the drug has been taken at night, food and smoking should be avoided, since both interfere with drug action. Treatment with H_2-receptor antagonists is usually only necessary for two or three months, especially if patients adopt a changed lifestyle. Relapses will occur especially if patients eat late meals. If recurrences are frequent or persistent, or if the oesophagitis is severe, patients may require long-term, continuous treatment with H_2-receptor antagonists. Although continuous treatment may be a nuisance to patients, it presents no health risks as the H_2-receptor antagonists are remarkably safe.

Some patients do not respond satisfactorily to H_2-receptor antagonists alone and may then benefit if the drug is combined with a prokinetic drug such as cisapride (pages 46–7). Cisapride is also given two to four times daily and complements the acid inhibition of the H_2-receptor antagonist drug by improving the function of the oesophageal muscles. Such treatment may have to be continued for many months or even years.

Proton pump inhibitors

More recently, some very powerful inhibitors of gastric acid secretion, called proton pump inhibitors (omeprazole and lansoprazole) (see page 48), have been used to treat oesophagitis. Because these drugs are more powerful than H_2-receptor antagonists, they can be used to treat patients whose oesophagitis is not healed, and when complaints are not controlled by H_2-receptor antagonists. Proton pump inhibitors are often very effective in controlling indigestion and heartburn in these patients.

However, treatment for oesophagitis often has to be long term because stopping treatment may be followed rapidly by the return of symptoms. The long-term safety of proton pump inhibitors is still under investigation. Operations are therefore often used as treatment.

Endoscopic treatment

When a doctor finds that, in addition to oesophagitis, the patient suffers from a complication such as narrowing of the oesophagus, the narrowed area has to be stretched.

Nowadays, this is often done by passing a thin tube with a deflated balloon down a channel in the endoscope. Once inside the narrowed oesophagus, the balloon is inflated and the narrowed segment of the oesophagus is gently stretched.

The procedure is repeated with balloons of increasing size until the passage is widened satisfactorily.

This procedure may have to be repeated at a later date, but satisfactory treatment with a gastric acid inhibitor slows down the scarring caused by further exposure to regurgitated gastric juice.

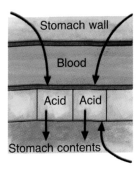

H_2-receptor antagonists

Prostaglandins

Stomach wall

Blood

Acid   Acid

Stomach contents

Proton pump blockers

Site of action of gastric acid inhibitors.

Surgery

A few patients will need an operation to reconstruct and tighten the lower end of the oesophagus and to repair an hiatal hernia. The operation is now often performed as 'key hole' surgery so that the patient need only spend one or two days in hospital. The risks from this operation are low, complications are uncommon, and the results are satisfactory in the majority of patients.

OUTLOOK

Although oesophagitis is a nuisance because of symptoms such as heartburn, it is a harmless condition that does not affect survival. Only a very small proportion of patients (1–2%) develop scarring of the lower oesophagus and difficulty in swallowing food.

Inflammation of the lining of the oesophagus is often difficult to heal completely because the underlying flabbiness of the muscles at the lower end of the oesophagus cannot easily be corrected except by surgery. However, the symptoms caused by oesophagitis can usually be kept under control by change in lifestyle and by taking drugs that inhibit gastric acid secretion and those that improve muscle function.

KEY POINTS

Symptoms of oesophagitis
- ✓ Regurgitation, heartburn, pain, difficulty in swallowing, bleeding, chronic cough and chronic laryngitis

Investigations
- ✓ Endoscopy, barium meal X-rays, measurement of acidity in oesophagus and measurement of movement of food through oesophagus

Treatment
- ✓ Lifestyle changes, raft antacids, prokinetic drugs, gastric acid inhibitors or surgery

Outlook
- ✓ Oesophagitis is a chronic nuisance, but usually does not interfere with health. Complaints can generally be controlled by changing lifestyle and by use of simple drug treatments during flare-ups

Gastric and duodenal ulcers

Duodenal ulcers are more common than gastric ulcers and occur especially in younger individuals. Early during this century, men were much more often affected by duodenal ulcers than women, but the frequency in women has now caught up – perhaps because of the recent increase in smoking among women. There are often considerable differences in the occurrence of duodenal ulcers within countries. In the UK,

GASTRIC AND DUODENAL ULCERS

Gastric and duodenal ulcers are small, round or oval wounds in the lining of the stomach and duodenum, respectively.

These ulcers are common and occur in about one in ten of the population.

for example, the disease becomes more common the further north one travels, with the highest rate in Scotland. Recently, gastric ulcers have become more common, especially in elderly patients and particularly in women older than 60 years. People in this age group are more likely to need drug treatment for conditions such as arthritis and rheumatism and this type of treatment is probably the major cause of gastric ulcers.

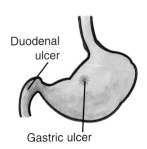

Duodenal ulcer

Gastric ulcer

Location of gastric and duodenal ulcers.

CAUSES OF ULCERS

Acid

It is not known what causes either type of ulcer but the most widely held view is that they are caused by over-production of gastric juice. Gastric juice secreted by the stomach contains strong hydrochloric acid and a ferment called 'pepsin' that breaks down the proteins of meat, milk, etc. The pepsin only works under acidic conditions and, therefore, the mixture of acid and pepsin makes a very powerful erosive combination. When too much gastric acid is discharged into the duodenum, the affected individual may develop a duodenal ulcer. Substantial reduction of the secretion of acid and pepsin, using drugs that inhibit gastric secretion, is usually sufficient to heal duodenal ulcers. However, some patients with gastric or duodenal ulcers produce normal amounts of gastric juice so that other causes for the ulcer have been sought.

Diet

It has been suggested that eating too much salt may cause gastric ulcers. Coffee and cola drinks are stimulants of gastric secretion and their excessive consumption by young people has been linked with the development of duodenal ulcers later in life. Lack of roughage does not cause ulcers but increases the likelihood of relapse in individuals who have previously suffered from ulcer disease.

Smoking

Smoking impairs the healing of ulcers and promotes the relapse of healed ulcers. Smoking also interferes with the action of some anti-ulcer drugs.

Drugs

The use of aspirin and antirheumatic drugs is associated with the development of gastric and duodenal ulcers. The drugs injure the lining of the stomach and duodenum very rapidly. Maximal injury occurs during the first week of treatment but then improves. However, as the inflammation decreases, an ulcer may develop. It has been estimated that approximately one quarter of patients receiving continuous treatment with aspirin or antirheumatic drugs develop an ulcer during the course of the treatment. These ulcers are more dangerous than ordinary ulcers since they often do

CAUSES OF ULCERS

- Gastric acid and pepsin
- Diet
- Smoking
- Aspirin and other antirheumatic drugs
- *Helicobacter pylori* infection

not produce pain or indigestion but, instead, show themselves with an ulcer complication such as bleeding.

Infection

It has been suggested that factors in the environment may cause ulcers. Among the possible culprits are infectious agents. During the past ten years, it has been suggested that a bacterium, called *Helicobacter pylori*, is the cause of ulcers. This bacterium lives in the stomach between the lining and its protective covering of mucus. In the Western world, the likelihood of infection increases with increasing age. In less developed countries, most individuals are infected – often from early childhood. The bacterium is found not only in the stomach but also in dental plaque and in the stools. Infection with *Helicobacter pylori* seems to occur in childhood and less commonly in adult life.

Only a small proportion of the infected individuals ever develop an ulcer. It is not known what features of the bacterium or the patient determine who develops an ulcer and who does not. The most important evidence for the involvement of *Helicobacter pylori* in causing ulcers relates to the treatment of the infection with antibiotics, because antibacterial drugs not only eradicate the infection, but heal the ulcers and keep them healed for many months.

SYMPTOMS

Pain in the central upper abdomen just under the breast bone is the most common complaint and affects almost all patients. Patients with gastric ulcers have often suffered from pain for a shorter period of time (less than one year) than patients with duodenal ulcers who have usually complained of pain on and off for many years. Other less common symptoms include nausea and vomiting. The vomiting usually relieves the ulcer pain.

The pain of duodenal ulcers is usually eased by eating and by antacid preparations although in some patients, especially those with gastric ulcers, food may actually make the pain worse. With duode-

---

SYMPTOMS OF ULCER DISEASE

Gastric ulcer
- Pain less than one year
- Pain aggravated by food
- Loss of appetite
- Nausea and vomiting

Duodenal ulcer
- Pain for many years
- Pain sharply localized in upper abdomen
- Pain relieved by food
- Pain wakes patient at night
- Vomiting relieves pain

nal ulcers, even if eating does provide temporary relief, the pain often returns 20–30 minutes after the meal. The pain of duodenal ulcers is localized and can often be pointed to with one finger. In addition, the pain of a duodenal ulcer characteristically wakes the patient at night. Loss of appetite occurs in approximately two-thirds of gastric ulcer patients. If therefore a patient suffers daily pain that is brought on by eating and is accompanied by loss of appetite, the ulcer is more likely to be gastric than duodenal, especially if the patient is elderly and taking antirheumatic pills.

COMPLICATIONS OF ULCER DISEASE

Sometimes ulcers do not cause pain. These 'silent' ulcers, which are most common in individuals who have been taking antirheumatic drugs, often persist for some time without giving rise to any trouble and may then heal by themselves. However, in some patients, the ulcer may show its presence by giving rise to a complication.

There are two main complications – bleeding and perforation – and one that is much less common called 'pyloric stenosis'. Bleeding from an ulcer usually causes vomiting of blood or the passage of black, tar-like stools. Bleeding ulcers re-

quire treatment in hospital. Perforation means that the ulcer has eroded its way through the entire thickness of the wall of the stomach or duodenum so that the contents of these organs can leak into the abdominal cavity. The perforation causes sudden intense abdominal pain and the patient becomes very ill and has to go to hospital immediately. Pyloric stenosis (narrowing) is the name given to the scarring around a healed duodenal ulcer, usually after many episodes of recurrence and rehealing, The scarring results in obstruction to the exit from the stomach at the pylorus. Pyloric stenosis causes repeated vomiting that can only be resolved surgically or by stretching the narrowed area.

COMPLICATIONS OF ULCER DISEASE

Haemorrhage
- Vomiting blood
- Tarry black stools

Perforation
- Severe generalized abdominal pain
- Requires urgent admission to hospital

Pyloric stenosis
- Repeated persistent vomiting
- Weight loss

TESTS AND INVESTIGATIONS

The diagnosis of ulcer disease must always be confirmed endoscopically. Endoscopy is undoubtedly the best investigation for confirming the diagnosis of gastric or duodenal ulcer because the doctor can actually see exactly where the ulcer is, its size and whether it is bleeding. A barium meal X-ray is not as good since this test fails to detect up to one third of ulcers. Whenever a gastric ulcer is found during endoscopy or on barium X-ray, it is always necessary to obtain some small pieces of the lining of the ulcer (biopsy specimens) for examination under a microscope, as the stomach ulcer may be cancerous.

In addition, nowadays the doctor who carries out the endoscopy also usually takes several little pieces of tissue from the lining of the stomach so that they can be looked at under a microscope and sent to the laboratory for bacterial culture, to see whether the patient is infected with *Helicobacter pylori*.

Infection with *Helicobacter pylori* can also be confirmed by carrying out a blood test, which may show evidence of the infection. Alternatively, the individual may be asked to undergo a very simple and completely harmless 'urea breath test'. In this test, the patient is asked to swallow some water that contains

INVESTIGATIONS OF ULCER DISEASE
● Endoscopy
● Biopsy
● Barium meal X-ray
● *Helicobacter pylori* tests
Microscopy of biopsy specimen
Culture of biopsy specimen
Blood tests
Urea breath tests

a small amount of urea, a substance that we all have circulating in our blood. The *Helicobacter pylori* bacteria are able to break down the urea into carbon dioxide and water. Carbon dioxide is a gas that we all normally produce in the body and which we breathe out from our lungs. In the test, the carbon atom of the urea is altered so that it 'labels' the carbon dioxide into which the urea is broken down. The patient breathes into a container in which there is fluid that can trap the carbon dioxide which is breathed out. It is therefore possible to measure how much of the labelled urea has been broken down. If patients are infected with *Helicobacter pylori* in the stomach, quite a lot of labelled carbon dioxide appears, while in uninfected individuals, there is virtually none.

When endoscopy is not readily

available, the doctor may request a barium meal X-ray (see page 19). Barium X-rays are not the primary choice of investigation because they do not provide as much, or as certain, information as endoscopy.

TREATMENT

Drug treatment

Patients with ulcers are at risk from the twin complications of bleeding and perforation, so priority has to be given to healing the ulcer. We now have available two principal means of treating ulcers.

Firstly, we can use drugs that block the production of acid by the stomach. The H_2-receptor antagonists (see page 47) have been shown to heal eight out of 10 ulcers within four weeks of the start of treatment, while most of the remainder heal after another month or two of treatment. In addition, the pain associated with the ulcer is usually relieved within 48 hours of starting the treatment and, while the ulcer is healing, the patients are no longer at risk from complications.

The few ulcers that do not heal may be treated with a combination of a gastric acid inhibitor and antibacterial drugs (see page 32) or, if that form of treatment also fails, can be treated surgically after investigation to exclude some very rare diseases that cause ulcers.

Occasionally, doctors use other drugs to heal ulcers including a group of drugs called prostaglandins. Misoprostol (*Cytotec*) is one example. These drugs are weak inhibitors of gastric acid secretion and their effect on ulcer healing and remission is not as good as with the H_2-receptor antagonists. However, it has been claimed that misoprostol protects the stomach lining against antirheumatic drugs and it may be used when antirheumatic drugs are essential. Sometimes the very powerful inhibitors of gastric secretion, called proton pump inhibitors (see page 48) are used because these drugs heal ulcers faster than do the H_2-receptor antagonists. Alternatively, some doctors prefer antacids or preparations that are called 'mucosal protective' drugs, such as sucralfate or a bismuth-containing preparation. These drugs coat the ulcer and are thought to stop the injurious effects of acid and pepsin. Usually, these other types of treatment have no advantage over H_2-receptor antagonists for healing ulcers.

Relapses

Unfortunately, more than eight out of ten ulcers healed with inhibitors of acid secretion or mucosal protective drugs relapse within one year of treatment and about half of the patients treated in that way relapse twice or more in a year. A first

TREATMENT OF GASTRIC AND DUODENAL ULCERS

The treatment of gastric and duodenal ulcers is virtually identical. The patient must not take aspirin or antirheumatic drugs (also known as non-steroidal anti-inflammatory drugs), unless this treatment is absolutely essential. The patient should stop smoking, since smoking delays the healing of ulcers and encourages relapses. No special diet is necessary but ulcer patients should ensure that they eat a well-balanced diet containing sufficient roughage and vitamins.

relapse may be treated like the original episode of ulcer disease. However, since any recurrence of an ulcer can be accompanied by a complication, especially if there has been a haemorrhage or perforation previously, or if the patient has received antirheumatic drugs, in most patients treatment must be designed to keep ulcers healed. That objective can be achieved by using long-term continuous treatment with H₂-receptor antagonists.

Long-term treatment

Continuous long-term treatment with H₂-receptor antagonists is the most satisfactory way of dealing with recurrent ulcers. The drug is taken every night for many years During continuous treatment, the H₂-receptor antagonist acts as a blanket on smouldering coals and prevents the flames of ulcer relapse from flickering. If treatment is stopped at any time, even for a few days, the ulcer may recur. Consequently, patients should not

(and from experience, do not) forget their pills when they go on holiday.

Relapses during long-term treatment

Long-term treatment works well for most patients but in a few, especially heavy smokers and patients taking antirheumatic drugs, relapses occur during the first year or two after healing in spite of continuous treatment. The recurrences are harmless and often do not cause pain. These ulcers are easily re-healed by doubling the dose of H₂-receptor antagonist. After re-healing, long-term treatment should be continued at a bigger dose.

Duration of long-term treatment

Patients whose ulcers stay healed during the first year of long-term treatment will usually have no further problems as long as treatment is continued.

Unfortunately, however long the treatment, it seems at present that eighty per cent of these patients will have a relapse if treatment is stopped. Therefore long-term treatment must be continued for many years and perhaps even for life. Although it may be a nuisance, long-term treatment with H_2-receptor antagonists is very safe and side effects are exceptionally rare.

Antibacterial treatment

Based on the assumption that ulcers are caused by infection with *Helicobacter pylori*, it has recently been proposed that all ulcer patients should receive a course of antibacterial drugs as the first choice of treatment. What this means is that every patient who is suspected of having an ulcer should have the diagnosis confirmed by endoscopy. If an ulcer is present, the patient should receive antibacterial treatment.

Antibiotic combinations

In order to get rid of (eradicate) the infection with *Helicobacter pylori*, it is essential to use combinations of antibacterial drugs. At least three components seem to be necessary (see page 50).

Problems with antibacterial treatment

The combination of antibacterial drugs is difficult to take because it involves swallowing at least eight tablets, and often more, and at least two tablets have to be taken four times daily for one or two weeks. Many patients find that sort of schedule inconvenient, or just do not remember to take the drugs. Elderly patients with an ulcer find this sort of treatment especially confusing because, unless the tablets are well organized and labelled, it may be difficult to remember what has, or has not, been taken.

Combination treatment has side effects, which range from inconvenient to severe.

As a result of the side effects, about five per cent of patients do

SIDE EFFECTS OF COMBINATION TREATMENT

- Diarrhoea
- Nausea
- Vomiting
- Abdominal pain
- Metallic taste
- Sore mouth
- Thrush (mouth or vagina)
- Itching
- Rash

not complete the course and the treatment may then be unsuccessful. Another problem is that the treatment does not heal the ulcers of about one in ten patients who do take the course.

Outcome of antibacterial treatment

The most impressive result of

THE THREE COMPONENTS OF ANTIBACTERIAL TREATMENT

1. Either a gastric secretory inhibitor (such as the proton pump inhibitor omeprazole or an H_2-receptor antagonist such as ranitidine) or a preparation containing bismuth, such as colloidal bismuth subcitrate (*De-Nol*)
2. An antibiotic such as amoxycillin, tetracycline or clarithromycin
3. An antibacterial drug such as metronidazole

antibacterial treatment of ulcers is that relapse of the ulcers is much delayed or prevented for at least a year or two in the majority of patients whose infection has been eradicated. It is this aspect of antibacterial treatment with a combination of drugs that has led a group of gastroenterology experts recently to recommend that all patients with proven ulcers should receive a course of antibacterial treatment.

There remain a few outstanding problems. There is no agreement yet on the best type of combination of antibiotics to be used for the treatment. If the treatment does not eradicate the infection, many of the ulcers relapse. Similarly, patients who are reinfected may relapse. The best treatment of relapse is uncertain at present but these patients do, of course, respond very well to continuous treatment with H_2-receptor antagonist drugs, as do patients whose ulcers do not heal with, or who cannot manage, or tolerate, the antibacterial treatment. One further

group of patients requires special consideration – patients whose ulcers have been caused by antirheumatic drugs. This type of ulcer may heal with antibacterial treatment but tends to relapse, even in the absence of infection with *Helicobacter pylori* bacteria. Since recurrence of ulcers caused by antirheumatic drugs is potentially dangerous, because so many of these patients suffer from ulcer complications, patients with ulcers caused by antirheumatic drugs should receive long-term continuous treatment with H_2-receptor antagonists.

Surgical treatment

In the UK, surgery is no longer used for the treatment of uncomplicated ulcer disease because operations are followed by irreversible complications in quite a number of patients. The most common operations performed in ulcer patients included gastrectomy (removal of part of the stomach) or vagotomy (cutting the vagus nerves to the stomach, which control acid production). Today, surgery is usually only undertaken in patients whose ulcers do not heal with drug treatment or in those whose occupations make reliable, long-term drug treatment impossible (for example, sailors and those working abroad in remote places). Surgical treatment may also be necessary to treat the complications of ulcer disease.

OUTLOOK

During the past few years, ulcer treatment has been revolutionized and treatment of ulcers no longer presents a clinical problem. More than ninety five per cent of ulcers can be healed and the majority can be kept healed, although the best way to achieve permanent remission is still being studied. Antibacterial treatment is very promising but has not been available long enough to establish the long-term outlook. On the other hand, with H_2-receptor antagonists, it is now possible to heal ulcers easily and keep them healed, so that patients who continue to take their tablets are restored to normal health.

KEY POINTS

Symptoms of gastric and duodenal ulcers
✓ Pain, nausea, vomiting and haemorrhage

Investigations
✓ Endoscopy, biopsy, barium meal X-ray, blood tests and breath tests

Treatment
✓ Stop smoking, avoid aspirin and antirheumatic drugs if possible, take drugs that inhibit gastric acid secretion or drugs that eradicate *Helicobacter pylori* infection

Outlook
✓ The majority of ulcer patients can be restored to normal health

Stomach (gastric) cancer

Cancer is an uncontrolled growth of cells that will, if not stopped, spread locally or to other parts of the body. It seems likely that cancer of the stomach (gastric cancer) is caused by environmental factors. The most interesting evidence for this comes from migrant studies. For example, gastric cancer is very common in Japan. The Japanese who migrate to the USA have almost as much gastric cancer as those remaining in Japan, but the children of the immigrants show a decrease in frequency to that found among the local US population. It seems, therefore, that the cause of gastric cancer in Japan is related to environmental influences early in life. Among the foodstuffs that have been implicated are pickled vegetables and smoked or salted meat and fish. Conversely, a diet containing milk and fresh vegetables is thought to protect against this type of cancer.

HOW COMMON IS GASTRIC CANCER?

Gastric cancer is encountered especially among poorer people, in men rather than women, and among those in the age group 50–70 years. Gastric cancer is also more common in patients who are heavy drinkers. There is also an increased likelihood of developing gastric cancer in patients who have undergone gastrectomy or who are suffering from pernicious anaemia (an inherited disease, which results in atrophy, or thinning, of the stomach lining and in anaemia because the patients cannot absorb vitamin B_{12} from their food). It has recently been suggested that chronic long-term

GASTRIC CANCER

Cancer of the stomach has become less common in the UK during the past 30 years.

infection with the bacterium *Helicobacter pylori* increases the likelihood of developing cancer of the stomach later in life.

SYMPTOMS

It has been estimated that less than one in 100 patients who seek advice for indigestion are suffering from gastric cancer. A history of recent onset of indigestion in a patient older than 50 years should, however, always arouse suspicion of gastric cancer, particularly if the pain or discomfort is continuous and is accompanied by loss of appetite, vomiting and weight loss. The pain of gastric cancer is often severe and is not related to eating and is made worse by food. The pain may be relieved by antacids at first. Obvious bleeding is not common but anaemia is frequently found.

TESTS AND INVESTIGATIONS

Any of the above symptoms in a patient over 50 years of age requires early endoscopic examination to determine whether there is a gastric ulcer or tumour. If there is, biopsy specimens will be taken for microscopic examination to confirm or exclude the diagnosis of cancer.

TREATMENT

Gastrectomy, with removal of part or all of the stomach, is the only form of treatment that can cure the disease and, if treated early enough, about eight in 10 patients survive normally for many years. Unfortunately, gastric cancer is often not diagnosed until it is quite far advanced.

Radiotherapy (treatment with X-rays) will not produce a cure but may be useful for controlling unpleasant symptoms in some patients. Drug therapy (chemotherapy) is also useful in some patients.

Gastrectomy

This operation can either remove part of the stomach (partial gastrectomy) or all of it (total gastrectomy). After the operation, the patient is fed through a tube but within a few days the digestive tract has usually recovered sufficiently for the patient to begin eating and drinking again. The usual hospital stay is 10–14 days. After the operation patients are advised to eat frequent, small meals to avoid feeling distended. Patients must receive monthly injections of vitamin B_{12} since this vitamin cannot be absorbed properly after gastrectomy.

OUTLOOK

If diagnosed early, the outlook for patients is very good. The course of gastric cancer tends to be worse in young adults and in elderly patients; when there is difficulty in swallowing or a lot of vomiting; or if the cancer has spread to other parts of the body.

KEY POINTS

Symptoms of gastric cancer
- ✓ Pain, loss of appetite, vomiting, difficulty in swallowing, weight loss and anaemia

Investigations
- ✓ Endoscopy with biopsy

Treatment
- ✓ Surgery or chemotherapy. Radiotherapy for control of symptoms

Outlook
- ✓ Satisfactory if diagnosed early

Gastritis

ometimes gastric inflammation is sufficiently severe to produce little superficial ulcers (erosions) of the lining. In some patients, the inflammation progresses to thinning (atrophy) of the stomach lining, with loss of the glands that secrete acid and pepsin.

The likelihood of developing gastritis increases with age. This may be because infection with *Helicobacter pylori* is more common in older people or because older people take more antirheumatic drugs.

GASTRITIS

Gastritis is the name given to inflammation and/or thinning of the lining of the stomach. Chronic inflammation may be caused by infection with the bacterium *Helicobacter pylori* and by drugs (such as aspirin and other antirheumatic agents).

SYMPTOMS

Most patients suffering from gastritis have no complaints and do not suffer from any apparent ill health. Neither infection with *Helicobacter pylori* nor gastric inflammation gives rise to any symptoms. Occasionally, there is indigestion and flatulence.

If there are little ulcers of the stomach lining, these may produce upper abdominal pain.

TESTS AND INVESTIGATIONS

The stomach looks red and inflamed during endoscopic examination. Microscopic examination of a biopsy specimen shows the presence of inflammation and there is usually infection with *Helicobacter pylori*. Infection can be confirmed by a number of other tests, including bacterial culture of the biopsy specimen or a urea breath test.

TREATMENT

If the gastritis is caused by *Helicobacter pylori* infection, the condition can be treated with a combination of antibacterial drugs (page 50).

OUTLOOK

Successful eradication of the *Helicobacter pylori* infection results in the clearance of inflammation in many patients. However, the atrophy (thinning) of the stomach lining may persist.

KEY POINTS

Symptoms of gastritis
- ✓ Most patients have no complaints. Occasionally there may be indigestion or pain in upper abdomen

Investigations
- ✓ Endoscopy with biopsy and tests for *Helicobacter pylori* infection

Treatment
- ✓ Antibacterial treatment

Outlook
- ✓ Inflammation easily cleared. Thinning of stomach lining is often progressive

Non-ulcer dyspepsia

How common is non-ulcer dyspepsia?

Indigestion lasting longer than two weeks is a common cause of disability. A study undertaken in the north-east of Scotland showed that twenty-five per cent of patients visiting their GP suffered from this problem. Examination of sickness certificates in Sweden showed that indigestion without cause was the reason given for one in six absences from work. Non-ulcer dyspepsia accounts for about one half of the patients consulting their GP for indigestion. The proportion is higher in patients less than 45 years old, because approximately two-thirds of older patients with indigestion are found to be suffering from an identifiable disease.

Symptoms

In patients with indigestion, some patterns of complaints suggest that an individual is suffering from non-ulcer dyspepsia. For example, the person remains well and does not lose weight. He or she is hungry, but during meals is quickly full up. The individual suffers from regurgitation, bloating, flatulence and distension. Pain is present in eighty per cent of patients and is felt all over the abdomen. The pain is often present every day but not at night. There may be associated nausea and when the patient vomits, he or she cannot face food. There is often intolerance for lots of different foods.

NON-ULCER DYSPEPSIA

When no cause for the indigestion can be found (because the patient does not have endoscopic evidence of an ulcer or oesophagitis) the patient is considered to be suffering from 'non-ulcer dyspepsia'

SYMPTOMS OF NON-ULCER DYSPEPSIA

- Pain felt all over abdomen
- Pain present every day but not at night
- No weight loss
- Regurgitation, bloating & flatulence
- Intolerance to many different foods

The pattern of symptoms in patients suffering from non-ulcer dyspepsia can be divided into three main groups:

1. Ulcer-like indigestion: The pattern of pain and symptoms is typical of ulcer disease but no ulcer can be found after thorough testing.

2. Reflux-like indigestion: Symptoms suggest the presence of oesophagitis but there is no endoscopic evidence of oesophageal disease.

3. Indigestion caused by 'dysmotility': This type of indigestion is associated with abnormal muscular function of the stomach and small intestine, so that food and gas are not moved along normally (dysmotility) but are shuttled back and forth, or there may simply be too little movement. This type of indigestion is also called 'flatulent' indigestion, with flatulence, bloating, distension and an early 'full-up' feeling

when eating. However, on investigation, no pattern of movement disturbance is associated with any set of complaints. In some patients, there may be altered perception of gut volume, so that normal amounts of gas or food produce an abnormal sensation of fullness.

TESTS AND INVESTIGATIONS

It is important in patients with chronic indigestion to exclude the presence of identifiable disease, because if disease is present, its identification permits specific treatment. On the other hand, if no disease can be demonstrated, the patients can be greatly helped by reassurance and explanation. Under these circumstances, patients can usually cope with their complaints.

A series of investigations and tests are therefore usually carried out if complaints have been present for a month or more.

In patients with non-ulcer dyspepsia, endoscopic examination (page 15) shows no abnormality, so patients can be reassured about the absence of cancer of the stomach. If endoscopy is normal, further investigation is often not necessary.

During endoscopy, the lining of the oesophagus, stomach and duodenum are usually examined by taking some small pieces with a biopsy forceps for examination under a microscope. If the biopsy shows inflammation of the oesophagus, the diagnosis of oesophagitis is confirmed despite normal endoscopic appearances. Microscopic examination of the stomach lining can show inflammation and infection with the bacterium *Helicobacter pylori*, while microscopic examination of the lining of the duodenum may confirm the diagnosis of coeliac disease (which reflects an allergic response to wheat and rye products).

Tests for establishing the diagnosis of infection with *Helicobacter pylori* are described on page 29. If infection is present, it may account for the patient's complaints.

Sometimes an ultrasound investigation is necessary to confirm a diagnosis. Ultrasound involves bouncing high frequency sound waves through the region below the right ribs, because if there are gall stones present, these reflect the sound waves (like submarines reflect the sound waves of sonar) and the disturbance of the sound waves can be photographed.

Blood tests are always carried out to make sure that there is no serious disease. For example, doctors test the blood for abnormally high concentrations of calcium, sugar or fat because abnormal values can indicate the presence of illnesses that produce indigestion.

A trial of treatment with a gastric acid inhibitor may be undertaken by a doctor because so many patients suffer from indigestion and investigations like endoscopy may have a long waiting list. Patients who improve during this short course of treatment may be spared the costs and inconvenience of further tests if the improvement lasts. Therapeutic trials are worth using in individuals younger than 45 years. However, if complaints do not improve quickly, or if the patient is older than about 50 years, early endoscopic examination is indicated. A therapeutic trial can also be used if the patient has previously suffered from an ulcer or oesophagitis, or if the complaints are very suggestive of these conditions. Under these circumstances, it is worth giving a patient a two-week course of an H_2-receptor antagonist, a proton pump inhibitor or cisapride. This type of test must not be carried out in individuals who have difficulty in swallowing, or who have lost a lot of weight, or who have bled or are anaemic, because these patients require urgent investigation. Alternatively, patients with ulcer-like indigestion can be given 1–2 weeks of treatment with a combination of antibacterial drugs because eradication of infection with *Helicobacter pylori* may improve the indigestion even if the individual does not have an ulcer.

Unfortunately, treatment trials are most likely to benefit patients with ulcer disease or oesophagitis. If there is recurrence of symptoms after the treatment is finished, the patient will require further investigation.

DRUG TREATMENT OF NON-ULCER DYSPEPSIA

The treatment of indigestion in patients with non-ulcer dyspepsia must be on the basis of trial and error. It is therefore worth using the following therapeutic schedules in turn.

Antacids and H$_2$-receptor antagonists

The treatment of indigestion depends on the assumption that gastric acid is responsible for the complaints. For this reason, antacids are the first choice of treatment and do, indeed, help control the complaints in about one-third of individuals. Patients whose complaints are helped for only a short time can be treated with a four-week course of an H$_2$-receptor antagonist. If the symptoms persist, or recur, the patient must have an endoscopic examination.

Antibacterial drugs

Alternatively, it is often assumed that because so many individuals suffer from infection with *Helicobacter pylori*, it is worth testing for the infection and treating the patient if infected (or even treating as if infected, without testing first). The combinations of antibacterial drugs that are necessary are described on page 50. Although no link has been

TREATMENT OF NON-ULCER DYSPEPSIA

- Change in lifestyle
  Reduce intake of alcohol, stop smoking and, if possible, avoid aspirin and antirheumatic drugs
- Avoid factors that promote regurgitation of stomach contents into the oesophagus
- Seek advice to control stress
- Drugs to eliminate *Helicobacter pylori* infection

found between infection with *Helicobacter pylori* and non-ulcer dyspepsia, it does seem that the treatment used for eradication of this organism may relieve the indigestion.

Drugs that regulate motility

Drugs that alter bowel movement (prokinetic drugs) help approximately two-thirds of patients with indigestion.

OUTLOOK

Indigestion usually continues on and off for many years. Often no cause is found despite thorough testing and the condition is then considered to be caused by a minor disturbance of the normal function of the gut. However, one to two per cent of patients suffering from non-ulcer dyspepsia develop an actual ulcer each year and about three times as many are found to be suffering from demonstrable oesophagitis, so that if symptoms persist or worsen, or if there is a change in the complaints, the tests must be carried out all over again.

KEY POINTS

Symptoms of non-ulcer dyspepsia
✓ Indigestion, pain, nausea, heartburn, flatulence and feeling of fullness

Investigations
✓ Endoscopy with biopsy, tests for *Helicobacter pylori* infection, blood tests and ultrasound

Treatment
✓ Lifestyle changes
  Avoidance of aspirin and antirheumatic drugs – if possible
  Gastric secretory inhibitors or antibacterial drug treatment

Outlook
✓ Indigestion usually continues on and off for many years but does not affect general health. A few patients may develop ulcer disease and others may develop oesophagitis

Drug treatment

Many of the drugs used in the treatment of indigestion have already been mentioned. This section provides further details about the more commonly used drugs.

DRUG TREATMENT

It is right that patients should know about the drugs that have been prescribed for them but it is not always easy to obtain this information from the name on the package or bottle, or from the package insert.

ANTACIDS

Antacids are usually the first line of treatment as they often relieve symptoms of ulcers, oesophagitis or non-ulcer dyspepsia. The antacid preparations, which are made up as flavoured thick chalky suspensions or tablets, work by neutralizing the acid produced by the stomach.

Antacids should be taken four or more times daily when symptoms occur or are expected – usually about an hour after meals and at bedtime. Liquid preparations may be a little more effective and quicker acting, but the tablet preparations are much more convenient to carry around.

It is not possible to list all of the antacid preparations that can be prescribed or bought from a chemist without a doctor's prescription. Indigestion sufferers should experiment with the various preparations available until they find one that is effective and has a pleasant taste.

Potential side effects

Consumption of large quantities of an antacid containing magnesium compounds may produce diarrhoea, while a lot of aluminium tends to be constipating (which is why they are often combined).

Calcium-containing preparations

are best avoided if antacids are going to be used for a long time, because too much calcium can cause kidney damage. Sodium bicarbonate also should not be used long-term, because it may cause water retention in the body (giving rise to swollen legs) and may aggravate high blood pressure.

Antacids can interfere with the absorption, and therefore the effectiveness, of other drugs, such as anticoagulants, heart drugs, anti-epileptic drugs, antibiotics, etc. These drugs should not be taken for at least one hour after an antacid. Patients with kidney disease should only take antacids after discussion with their GP. If in doubt, patients should consult their GP or pharmacist.

and alginic acid, which is made from seaweed. This combination makes the antacid float to the surface of the stomach contents. When the patient lies down or stoops, the antacid 'raft' enters the oesophagus first and acts as a sort of 'ball valve'. These preparations act best in the upright position. Drugs in this category include *Gaviscon*, *Gastrocote* and *Topal*.

Gaviscon and *Gastrocote* contain sodium bicarbonate and therefore their use should be discussed with the GP if the patient suffers from swollen legs or high blood pressure.

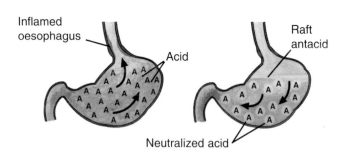

Raft antacids.

RAFT ANTACIDS

Raft antacids contain both an antacid

PROKINETIC DRUGS (MOTILITY STIMULANTS)

Prokinetic drugs are used in the treatment of oesophagitis and non-ulcer dyspepsia when motility problems seem to be causing the symptoms, that is, when the muscles which normally aid digestion fail to work properly.

The drugs can tighten the muscles around the lower end of the oesophagus, and stimulate the muscles that propel food and refluxed gastric contents out of the oesophagus and into the stomach. The drugs also improve muscle function in the stomach wall so that the stomach empties better into the intestine. There is also a general beneficial effect on the muscles in the wall of the intestine.

Drugs in this group include metoclopramide (*Maxolon*), domperidone (*Motilium*) and cisapride (*Prepulsid* or *Alimix*).

Potential side effects

Metoclopramide has a number of side effects, including drowsiness, diarrhoea and muscle spasms, which are more likely to occur in children than in adults. Alcohol may increase the sedative effects of the drug.

Domperidone may produce breast tenderness and menstrual irregularities.

Cisapride is now the drug of choice if a prokinetic agent is required for treatment. This drug improves motility along the whole length of the gut. The drug may give rise to abdominal cramps and diarrhoea. Very rarely, patients have reported headaches and convulsions.

H$_2$-RECEPTOR ANTAGONISTS

The H$_2$-receptor antagonists are a group of drugs so named because they block the effects of histamine on the stomach. Histamine is a hormone that is released in the stomach wall when food is eaten and then stimulates the secretion of gastric acid and pepsin.

The H$_2$-receptor antagonists heal gastric and duodenal ulcers by moderately reducing the amount of acid produced by the stomach. For the same reason they are also used in the treatment of oesophagitis, as well as in non-ulcer dyspepsia. The H$_2$-receptor antagonists should not be used for treating patients older than 50 years until a positive diagnosis has been made because the drugs may, by reducing symptoms, delay the diagnosis of gastric cancer.

The drugs in this group include cimetidine (*Tagamet*), ranitidine (*Zantac*), famotidine (*Pepcid*) and nizatidine (*Axid*).

Potential side effects

The H$_2$-receptor antagonists have been available for more than ten years and have been found to be remarkably safe when used continuously for the long-term treatment of ulcers and oesophagitis. Occasional side effects include a rash, diarrhoea, headache, drowsiness, or confusion in the elderly. By reducing the amount of acid in the stomach, the H_2-receptor antagonists may interfere with the absorption of some other drugs, such as antibiotics and iron preparations.

Cimetidine interferes with the functions of the liver that are responsible for breaking down other drugs. As a result, drugs such as anticoagulants, anti-epileptic drugs, beta-blockers for angina, sedatives, etc., may reach higher concentrations than normal in the blood and may then produce increased or prolonged effects. The dose of the other drugs may have to be decreased or, preferably, one of the other H_2-receptor antagonists should be used since they do not affect liver function appreciably. Large doses of cimetidine may also sometimes cause breast enlargement and impotence.

PROTON PUMP INHIBITORS

A number of these powerful suppressants of gastric acid production are currently being developed. These drugs act by stopping the acid-producing cells of the stomach from letting out their acid, so that the degree of gastric acid suppression is much more complete than with H_2-receptor antagonists, if the dose of the proton pump inhibitor is adequate. Omeprazole (*Losec*) has been available for nearly five years

and lansoprazole (*Zoton*) is now available for the treatment of ulcers and oesophagitis.

There is no real advantage in using proton pump inhibitors rather than H_2-receptor antagonists for the treatment of ulcers. However, because of their powerful gastric inhibitory action, these drugs are more effective than H_2-receptor antagonists in the treatment of oesophagitis. Unfortunately, in many patients, the symptoms of oesophagitis recur rapidly if treatment is stopped, so treatment must often be continuous and long-term.

Potential side effects

The side effects of omeprazole include headache, diarrhoea and skin rashes. Omeprazole may inhibit the liver function that breaks down other drugs so that use of omeprazole must be checked with the GP if the patient is taking drugs such as anticoagulants, anti-epileptic drugs or sedatives.

Long-term administration of omeprazole to rats has been shown to produce tumours in the stomach of treated animals. Although in the UK, official permission has been given for the long-term use of omeprazole in the treatment of ulcers or oesophagitis, surgical treatment may, at present, be a preferable option if oesophagitis cannot be controlled easily with drugs.

PROSTAGLANDINS

Prostaglandins are naturally-occurring, hormone-like substances that have been modified chemically to stop them from being broken down rapidly in the body. These drugs have two main actions on the stomach – they are weak inhibitors of gastric acid secretion and they are also thought to protect the lining of the stomach and duodenum. The only drug in this group that is currently available is misoprostol (*Cytotec*).

This drug is not much use in the treatment of ordinary ulcers but is claimed to be a satisfactory means for healing ulcers produced by antirheumatic drugs and also for protecting against the damage caused to the lining of the stomach and duodenum by antirheumatic drugs. The main role of misoprostol in ulcer treatment is therefore its use in patients who definitely require antirheumatic drugs for the treatment of severe joint disease.

Potential side effects

Diarrhoea may be severe and may require reduction in the dose of the drug. Patients may also suffer from abdominal pain, flatulence, nausea and vomiting. Misoprostol affects the muscles of the womb and may cause irregular or painful bleeding. Misoprostol should not be taken by pregnant women or those planning pregnancy.

MUCOSAL PROTECTIVE DRUGS

Sucralfate

Sucralfate (*Antepsin*) is a compound of aluminium and a sugar derivative that is thought to act by strengthening the lining of the oesophagus, stomach and duodenum, thereby increasing the resistance to damage by gastric acid and pepsin.

Potential side effects: Sucralfate may produce constipation, dry mouth and rashes. Other drugs, like anti-epileptic medications and digoxin, should not be given at the same time as sucralfate because their absorption may be decreased.

Bismuth compounds

Bismuth compounds alone can heal ulcers but these preparations are not popular for long-term use because bismuth can be very toxic to the nervous system. Recently, bismuth preparations – especially *DeNol* (which is colloidal bismuth subcitrate) – have been used in combination with antibiotics for treatment lasting one to two weeks.

Potential side effects: Bismuth compounds result in blackening of the tongue and stools. This discoloration is of no consequence.

COMBINATION TREATMENT

In order to eradicate infection with *Helicobacter pylori*, a number of combinations of drugs have been used (see table below). The best treatment combination has not yet been decided.

COMMONLY USED DRUG COMBINATIONS

- Bismuth, amoxycillin plus metronidazole
- Bismuth, tetracycline plus metronidazole
- Omeprazole plus amoxycillin
- Omeprazole, amoxycillin plus metronidazole
- Omeprazole, clarithromycin plus metronidazole
- Ranitidine, amoxycillin plus metronidazole

ANTIBIOTICS

Amoxycillin

Amoxycillin (*Amoxil* and other preparations) is a penicillin-type antibiotic that is given three or four times daily for one to two weeks, depending on the combination of drugs that is being employed.

Potential side effects: Side effects include diarrhoea and rashes, and occasionally more severe allergic reactions. Individuals suffering from penicillin allergy must not take amoxycillin but should take tetracycline or clarithromycin instead. Amoxycillin may interfere with the action of the contraceptive pill.

Tetracycline

Several preparations are available. Tetracycline is a widely used antibiotic. In combination with bismuth and metronidazole, a 14-day course of treatment gives excellent rates of eradication of *Helicobacter pylori* infection.

Potential side effects: Side effects include nausea, vomiting, diarrhoea and rashes. Tetracycline can reduce the effectiveness of oral contraceptives.

Clarithromycin

Clarithromycin (*Klaricid*) is a relatively new antibiotic which, given four times daily, can be used instead of amoxycillin.

Potential side effects: Side effects include nausea, vomiting, diarrhoea, abdominal pain, headaches and rashes.

Metronidazole

A number of preparations are available. Metronidazole is an antibiotic that is used to treat infection by bacteria and other organisms that do not respond well to other antibiotics. Metronidazole must be used in combination with other antibiotics and bismuth, or a gastric-secretory inhibitor, because if *Helicobacter pylori* is exposed to metronidazole alone, the bacterium rapidly develops resistance to the drug.

Potential side effects: The most common side effects of metronidazole are nausea, abdominal pain, unpleasant metallic taste in the mouth, furred tongue and loss of appetite. Occasionally, patients develop dizziness or numbness and tingling of the extremities.

Metronidazole may increase blood levels, and therefore the effects, of anticoagulants and antiepileptic drugs. Metronidazole may also produce a very severe reaction if alcohol is taken during treatment with the drug, including flushing, intense headache, palpitations, nausea, vomiting and, in severe cases, collapse.

KEY POINTS

Drug treatments for indigestion
- ✓ Antacids
- ✓ Raft antacids: *Gaviscon, Gastrocote, Topal*
- ✓ Prokinetic drugs (motility stimulants): *Maxolon, Motilium, Prepulsid*
- ✓ H$_2$-receptor antagonists: *Tagamet, Zantac, Pepcid, Axid*
- ✓ Proton pump inhibitors: *Losec, Zoton*
- ✓ Mucosal protective drugs: *Antepsin*
- ✓ Bismuth compounds: *DeNol*
- ✓ Antibacterial drug combinations

Conclusions

Indigestion is a very common problem which most people experience at some time and some individuals experience a great deal of the time.

The name 'indigestion' is given to a group of complaints that are sometimes produced by common illnesses but for which there is often no obvious cause. Some of the conditions that can result in indigestion, such as ulcers, are a potential threat to health. For this reason, patients with continuous or recurrent symptoms should always undergo full clinical examination and tests, so that the correct treatment can be given.

This helpful and reassuring book by Sigrid Burridge and Kenneth Wormsley describes the possible causes of indigestion, the tests undertaken to make a firm diagnosis and the various available treatments. However, medical treatment is not the whole story and the authors emphasize the importance of lifestyle on the health (and otherwise) of the digestive system and explain methods by which individuals can help to reduce their indigestion.

Question & Answers

Certain questions about indigestion are frequently asked by patients. These questions need to be answered to prevent patients worrying unnecessarily.

● I have developed indigestion. Is there anything I can do to help myself?

You will probably benefit from a change in lifestyle as shown in the chapter on page 4. You can easily try to treat yourself with antacids and/or acid-inhibiting drugs bought over the counter from the chemist. Even if the medicine is successful in relieving your symptoms, you should still tell your doctor in case you have a more serious underlying complaint which is temporarily being hidden by the treatment. The treatment of indigestion should always be shared care between yourself and your doctor.

● If I have pain or discomfort after eating, does it mean that I have indigestion?

Not necessarily, because sometimes a large meal can cause angina from heart disease. If you have any doubts, you should consult your doctor.

● Should my indigestion be treated?

You should always visit your doctor if your symptoms persist for more than a week or two. In addition, you should also consult your doctor if your symptoms are sudden or severe, or if your condition does not respond to medicines that you have bought from the chemist.

● Will my problems return if my indigestion is treated?

Perhaps, because some of the causes of indigestion persist despite treatment. Consequently, treatment may be required for many years. If your symptoms return after stopping treatment, it is worth seeing your doctor again.

● My indigestion continues despite treatment. Is this serious?

It could be, and this is why you should always seek medical help. Unfortunately, some of the diseases that produce indigestion are difficult to treat, either because the underlying problem is mechanical (as in oesophagitis) or because the cause is not known (as in non-ulcer dyspepsia).

If you are taking drugs prescribed by your doctor and your symptoms persist, it is usually because the drug has not been taken for long enough or the dosage needs to be increased. If your symptoms persist, you should always visit your doctor again.

Useful Addresses

British Digestive Foundation
3 St Andrews Place
Regents Park
London
NW1 4LB
Telephone: (0171) 224 2012

This charitable organization was founded to support research into diseases of the gut. The Foundation has leaflets and booklets about many diseases and disorders of the digestive system which are available to patients.

British Society of Gastroenterology
3 St Andrews Place
Regents Park
London
NW1 4LB
Telephone   (0171) 387 3534

Most British gastroenterologists (specialists in digestive diseases) belong to this Society.

GET

WELL

SOON.

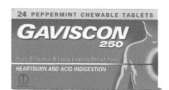

24 PEPPERMINT CHEWABLE TABLETS

GAVISCON 250

Fast, Effective & Long Lasting Relief from

HEARTBURN AND ACID INDIGESTION

HEARTBURN RELIEF

Index